THE FIFTY MINUTE

WORKOUT FOR PEOPLE

OVER FIFTY

by

GAILY WARREN

dp
DISTINCTIVE PUBLISHING CORP.

The Fifty Minute Workout for People Over Fifty
by Gaily Warren
Copyright 1993 by Gaily Warren

Published by Distinctive Publishing Corp.
P.O. Box 17868
Plantation, Florida 33318-7868
Printed in the United States of America

ISBN: 0-942963-25-3
Library of Congress No.: 92-18720
Price: $9.95

Library of Congress Cataloging-in-Publication Data

Warren, Gaily, 1949 -
   The fifty minute workout for people over fifty / Gaily Warren.
     p.   cm.
   Includes bibliographical references.
   ISBN 0-942963-25-3 : $9.95
   1. Exercise for the aged. 2. Physical fitness for the aged.
   I. Title.
   GV482.6.W37   1992
   613.7'0446—dc20   92-18720
                                        CIP

In memory of my parents,
George and Mary Warren.
I am grateful
that they shared their warmth,
positive spirit, kindness,
sense of humor, guidance
and love with me.

I miss them.

Personal Thanks
From The Author

I wish to thank, for their friendship, their labor and encouragement: Laura, Susan D., Susan L., Ceil, Denise, Kathy, Stella, Sally, Elaine, Barbra, Ted, Bill A., Bill B., Alan, and many other friends who helped me along the way.

Special Thanks

... to my brothers, Alex and Jig, for getting me involved in sports, our fun together, and the "special" friendship we share.

... to my husband, Todd, for your patience, love and belief in me.

... to my friends in all my classes, for their inspiration and giving back so much.

Table Of Contents

ABOUT THE AUTHOR ix

PREFACE xi

INTRODUCTION xiii

CHAPTER ONE: Chair Exercises 1

1. Warm-up 2

2. Isolations (Calisthenics) 3
   a. Legs and Feet 3
   b. Waist 4
   c. Arms, Chest, Shoulders, Upper Back 5

3. Aerobics 9

4. Isolations (Calisthenics) 11
   a. Leg Lifts 11
   b. Pelvic Squeezes (Kegels) .13
   c. Stomach 13

5. Cool-down Stretches 14
   a. Hands 14
   b. Arms, Shoulders, Chest, Upper Back 15
   c. Waist 15
   d. Legs, Stomach 16
   e. Body Roll 16

CHAPTER TWO: Water (Pool) Exercises 17

1. Warm-up: Aquatic Walking 18

2. Isolations (Calisthenics) 19
   a. Legs and Feet 19
   b. Waist 21
   c. Arms, Chest, Shoulders, Upper Back 22

3. Aerobics 24

4. Cool-down Walk 26

5. Wall Exercises: Isolations (Calisthenics) 26
   a. Stomach. 26
   b. Legs 27

6. Additional Wall Exercises 28
   a. Stomach. 28
   b. Buttocks, Upper Back or Legs 28

7. Cool-down Stretches. 28
   a. Legs, Feet, Stomach. 28
   b. Hands. 29
   c. Arms, Shoulders, Chest, Upper Back 29
   d. Waist 30
   e. Head Rolls 30

CHAPTER THREE: Indoor Standing
                  and Floor Exercises. 31

1. Warm-up. 32

2. Isolations (Calisthenics) 33
   a. Legs and Feet 33
   b. Waist 35
   c. Arms, Chest, Shoulders, Upper Back 36

3. Low-impact Aerobics 37

4. Cool-down Walk 39

5. Floor Exercises: Isolations (Calisthenics). 39
   a. Facial exercises. 40
   b. Push-ups 40
   c. Stomach. 41
   d. Outer Thighs. 42
   e. Inner Thighs 43
   f. Upper Front of Legs 44
   g. Buttocks, Upper Back of Legs 45

6. Cool-down Stretches 46
   a. Hands. 46
   b. Upper Back of Legs 46
   c. Lower Back. 47
   d. Shoulders. 47
   e. Head Rolls 47

BIBLIOGRAPHY. 49

ABOUT THE AUTHOR

THE AUTHOR OF *THE 50 MINUTE WORKOUT FOR PEOPLE OVER 50* was born in 1949. Reared in Sharon, Pennsylvania, she now lives in West Palm Beach, Florida, with her husband, Todd Eidenire.

Gaily Warren studied physical education, exercise physiology, nutrition and gerontology at the University of Tampa (Tampa, Florida) and Florida International University (Miami, Florida). Featured in south Florida by broadcast and print media for her exercise programs, she has participated throughout the country in numerous workshops related to exercise.

The author is a member of a number of professional organizations for fitness educators. Organizational memberships in her current home state include the Florida Adult and Community Educators, the Florida Adult Education Association, and the Professional Fitness of South Florida. Other groups which count her as a member are the REEBOK Professional Instructor Alliance, the International Dance Exercise Association, the NIKE Professional Instructor Association and the American College of Sports Medicine Association.

She works as an exercise instructor for the Adult and Community Education divisions of Dade County and Palm Beach County school systems. She also offers private instruction and has worked in corporate fitness.

Gaily Warren is certified as a Fitness Professional by the American Aerobics Association and the Institute of Aerobics Research.

PREFACE

I'VE ALWAYS LOVED TO EXERCISE. Growing up, I was happiest when swimming, bicycling, skiing or playing sports. As I grew older, I added calisthenics and exercise classes to my list of energizing activities.

After studying physical education in college, I went on to take additional courses in exercise physiology, gerontology, nutrition, and body composition. The more I expanded my knowledge of the effect exercise has on the body's general health, the more convinced I became that exercise is an essential key to feeling better—about oneself and life.

In 1983, I began teaching exercise classes in the Dade County School System's Adult Education Program. My courses included not only all different age groups, but also all different levels of physical ability.

To my surprise, I found working with older groups (people 50 and older) to be among the most interesting and satisfying of all my classes. At the beginning, however, I was alarmed at the physical condition of many of my students when I saw how difficult it was for them to so much as raise their arms or lift their legs. At other times I found myself amused. In the beginning, for example, the ladies came to class dressed in stockings, heels, skirts, jewelry and dress shirts and the men wore long pants with belts. Eventually, I was able to urge them into looser, more comfortable exercise clothes. Occasionally now, some show up in leotards, tights and workout shoes.

As I explained to them the benefits and pleasure of exercise and as they began to experience these for themselves, we all began to share in the joy of their results. I spent a lot of time listening to these older students, often asking them questions of my own. I carefully paced the program so that their classes would feel invigorating without being strenuous. After nine years, I am thrilled to see the ease with which my students now twist, bend, kick—and dance. Along with their increasing enthusiasm, their stamina also has grown.

My older students have taught me as much as I have taught them. I see how aging often is not easy. To me, however, my older students are living examples of how a consistent exercise program, coupled with a sense of humor, can enhance lifelong vitality.

INTRODUCTION

Each of the exercise routines in this book takes about fifty minutes to complete, at a leisurely pace. They have been specifically designed to improve cardiovascular tone and increase stamina and flexibility in people older than fifty years of age. The exercises are not strenuous. They do not demand enormous exertion or huge amounts of energy. You will find that all three chapters in this book use basically the same routine. They're just used a little differently according to where you are. Most important of all, they're meant to be fun!

Where to Exercise and What You'll Need

It's important to select a comfortable, well-ventilated part of your home for doing your exercises. You don't really need a lot of space, just enough to extend your arms and legs behind, to the side and in front of you without bumping or hitting anything. Also, you'll want enough floor space on which you can lie down and stretch out.

If you don't have an exercise mat (which can be purchased at any sporting goods or discount department store), you can use a towel.

For the chair exercises, any well-balanced, upright four-legged chair will work. It's possible for you to do these exercises from a folding chair, if it's steady and secure when open.

What to Wear

Loose, comfortable clothes lend themselves best to these exercises. While some people prefer to work out in leotards and tights, tee shirts, jogging shorts and even bathing suits are fine.

I suggest wearing socks and lace-up shoes with good arches, so that your feet, legs and back are well supported. Socks not only absorb perspiration, but also give additional support.

Music

Select whatever upbeat music you enjoy—big band, marching band, rhythm and blues, jazz, swing or rock 'n' roll—that is played at a tempo at which you can exercise and be comfortable.

Some examples of music you can use are:

Jazz — Najee, David Sanborn

Soul — Etta James, Luther Vandross

Rock 'n Roll — Rod Stewart, Buddy Holly

Big Band — Glenn Miller, Guy Lombardo

Movie Music — Out of Africa, Commitments

1

CHAIR EXERCISES

CHAIR EXERCISES

DOING EXERCISES FROM A CHAIR is for individuals who do not feel comfortable without a support system or those with physical limits. This can be a vigorous workout and quite a lot of fun. These exercises can be outside or inside. The ideal room temperature is 74°.

Warm-up

These exercises serve to slowly increase the heart rate and blood circulation, warm muscles, limber and lubricate joints and prepare the body for more demanding exercises and activities.

Sit tall in the middle of a chair (preferably one without arms), with feet flat on the floor. If sitting this way is uncomfortable on your back, sit back further in the chair.

Breathe. Take three deep breaths, inhaling through nostrils and inhaling slowly through mouth.

Warm up exercises:

Music should have an upbeat tempo but not too fast, lasting approximately three minutes.

1. Point the right toe, raise both arms in the air on right side; bring right foot back and point the left toe, lowering arms to waist. Do 12 times. Fig. 1.
2. Tap right heel, then left, alternating as both arms are pushing forward. Do 12 times. Fig. 2.

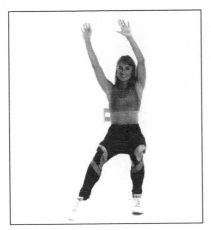
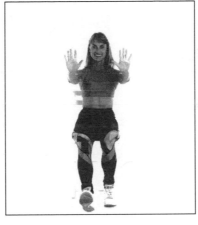
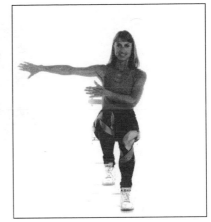

Fig 1   Fig 2   Fig 3

3. Lift right knee, then left, alternating knee lifts and taking both arms to right and then left according to the knee being lifted. You can vary this by moving arms to the opposite side of the knee lift. Do 12 times. Fig. 3.

4. Do this sequence for the length of the music chosen or at your individual discretion.

It should be noted that if an exercise does not feel comfortable, either it should be eliminated from the workout or repetitions should be decreased. Also, if a physically limited person is unable to exercise an arm or a leg, adapt the exercises to the capabilities.

Breathe. Take one deep breath, inhaling through nostrils and exhaling slowly through mouth.

Isolations (Calisthenics)

Legs and Feet

Music should have a beat which is somewhat slower than the Warm-up, running approximately three minutes. Listening to favorite songs makes the program more fun and enjoyable.

Sit tall.

1. Lift toes, both right and left for lower front leg strengthener. Do 12 times.

2. Lift heels both right and left for lower back leg strengthening. Do 12 times. Fig. 4.

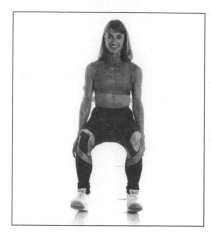

Fig 4

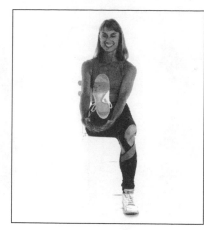

Fig 5

3. Raise right leg, holding it with one or both arms. Point toe, flex or flat foot. Do 12 times. Now change and do the same with left leg. Fig. 5.

4. Repeat the sequence for the length of the music or at your individual discretion.

5. Static or holding stretch: raise right leg, point toe, hold to a count of 12 and then flex or flat foot, hold to a count of 12.

   Breathe. Take one deep breath, inhaling through nostrils and exhaling slowly through mouth.

Waist

Music is same tempo for leg strengtheners.

1. With both arms at sides, shoulders back and feet flat on floor, lean slightly to right, extending arm halfway down leg of chair while left hand comes up to the waist. Do 12 times. Repeat sequence on left side. Fig. 6.

2. Hands on shoulders, head facing forward, turn to the right slightly and then to the left. Do 12 times. Fig. 7.

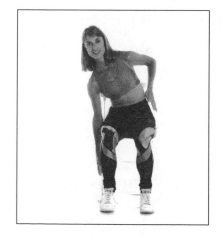

Fig 6

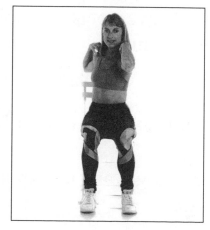

Fig 7

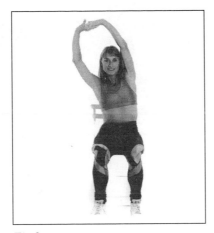

Fig 8

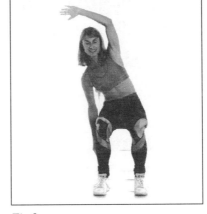

Fig 9

3. Raise both arms in the air, lace fingers. Move arms slightly to right and then to left. Do 12 times. Fig. 8.

4. Repeat entire sequence (1-3) for length of music or at your individual discretion.

5. Static or holding stretch: lean to right, holding front leg of chair with right hand, raising left arm overhead. Hold to a count of 12. Repeat on left side. Fig. 9.

Breathe. Take one deep breath, inhaling through nostrils and exhaling slowly through mouth.

Arms, Chest, Shoulders, Upper Back

Music tempo is a little more upbeat than the leg strengtheners and waist exercises.

It should be noted that for the following exercises, one can use hand weights, preferably one or two pounds each. Resistance without weights is used by pressing the air.

Upper front of arms:

1. Rest elbows on waist and bring forearms against chest, having hands cupped and pressing against the air. Pressing back against chair, lower arms, then raise them back to chest. Do 12 times. Fig. 10.

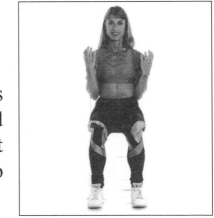

Fig 10

2. Extend arms to the front with forearms facing up and hands cupped. Bring cupped hands to shoulders pressing against the air. Do 12 times. Fig. 11.

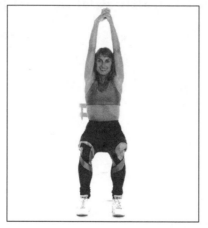

Fig 11

Upper back of arms:

1. With arms extended straight up, lace fingers and squeeze elbows to head. Take both arms behind head, as far down as possible, bending the elbows but keeping them close to the head, then raising arms in the air above head. Avoid over-extension into face area. Do 12 times. Figs. 12 & 13.

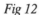

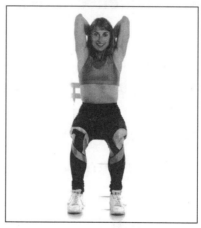

Fig 12   *Fig 13*

2. Place hands on each side of chest, make loose fists, bend elbows. Extend arms behind and then return fists to sides of chest. Do 12 times. Figs. 14 & 15.

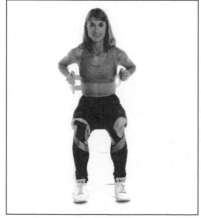   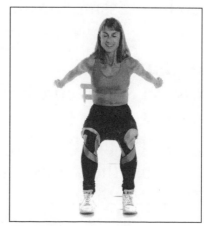

Fig 14   *Fig 15*

Chest and shoulders:

Bend both elbows with forearms extended in air on each side of chest. Bring both arms together, elbow to elbow, then back to the sides. Do 12 times. See Figs. 54 & 55, pg. 23.

Upper back and shoulders:

1. Extend arms straight out from sides, with loose fists. Bend elbows, bringing arms in front of chest, fists coming together. Do 12 times. Figs. 16 & 17.

2. Repeat sequence until music is finished or at your individual discretion.

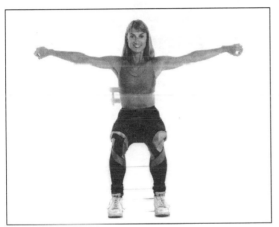

Fig 16

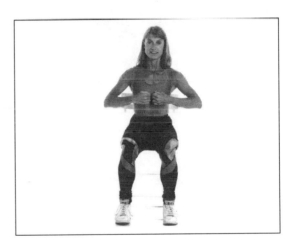

Fig 17

Static or holding stretches:

The following stretches can be done from a standing position or in a chair.

1. For upper back of arms and shoulders: Raise arms above head, dropping one arm behind head, placing one hand on opposite shoulder, other hand on elbow. Hold for a count of 12. Change arms and do the same for holding count of 12. Fig. 18.

2. For upper front of arms: Extend arms to sides with palms facing front and slightly toward back. Hold for a count of 12.

3. For upper back: Lace fingers behind back, raise arms and hold for a count of 12. Fig. 19.

4. For chest: Wrap arms around in front, give self a hug and hold for a count of 12.

5. Raise arms in air, and roll down as close to the floor as you can. Roll up slowly. Fig. 20.

6. Roll shoulders forward three times and backward three times. Fig. 21.

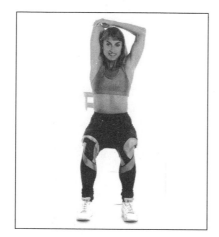

Fig 18

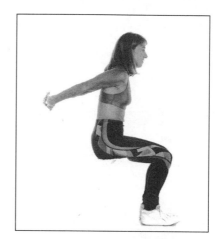

Fig 19

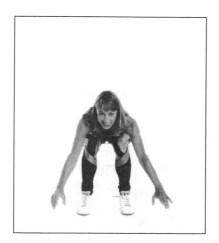

Fig 20

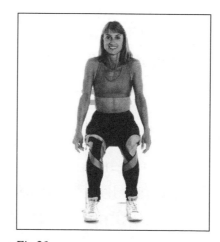

Fig 21

Aerobics

These exercises, which are geared to the cardio-respiratory system, strengthen the heart and lungs. Because the heart is a muscle, it requires exercise to keep it toned and healthy. The healthier the heart, the more efficiently the blood is pumped throughout the body. As the health of the lungs improves, the circulation of oxygen expands, and cells, tissues and muscles are better nourished. This builds endurance. Have a good time. Give 100%!

Music should have an upbeat tempo, beginning with a march and then getting faster. Use three or four different songs lasting ten to twenty minutes total.

Breathe. Take three deep breaths, inhaling through nostrils and exhaling slowly through mouth.

FIRST ROUTINE
March:

1. Lift knees up and down, bringing feet off the floor while alternating legs. Keep floor position of feet close together for count of 12. Repeat with feet further apart for count of 12. Vary the march. Swing arms with hands to opposite shoulders. Vary the arms as you march by orchestrating the arms, as though you are leading a band. Then raise arms in the air and wave. This can be performed in a standing position.

2. Repeat sequence until the music is finished or at your individual discretion.

SECOND ROUTINE

1. Lift knees while alternating legs. At the same time, raise arms and bring right elbow to left knee. Alternate with left elbow to right knee. Do 12 times. Fig. 22.

2. Push both legs and arms forward and back. Do 12 times.

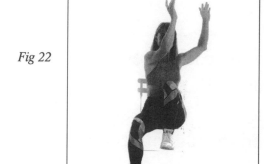

Fig 22

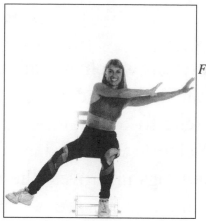

Fig 23

3. Kick legs to sides, one at a time, while pushing arms to opposite side of leg kick. Do 12 times. Fig. 23.

4. Repeat sequence until music is finished or at your individual discretion.

THIRD ROUTINE

1. Kick legs forward, one at a time. Simultaneously alternate arms, circling, as in the water crawl. Do 12 times. Fig. 24.

2. Tap heels while alternating legs. At the same time, push arms forward and then back to chest. Do 12 times. Fig. 25.

3. Kick legs to each side while swinging arms in the same direction. Do 12 times. Fig. 26.

4. Repeat sequence until music is finished or at your individual discretion.

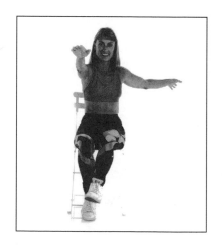

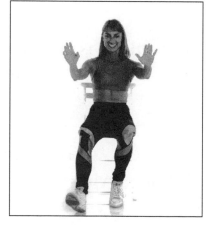

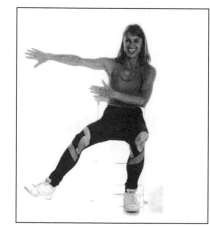

Fig 24   *Fig 25*   *Fig 26*

OTHER SUGGESTED ROUTINES

1. While lifting knees, hold hands above head, with elbows bent. Bring alternate elbow down as knee is lifted. Alternate sides and do 12 times.

2. Tap toes to front, alternating each leg while opposite arm is raised. Do 12 times.

3. *Modified jumping jack:* Alternate heel tapping on each side while arms are stretched out at sides. Raise arms in air, clapping hands overhead. Do 12 times.

4. *Beach ball throwing* (group activity): Ball is thrown between participants sitting in a circle. This is continued for length of song.

5. *Kick ball* with sponge ball (group activity): Participants sit in a circle and kick the ball to one another. This is continued for length of song.

Cool Down:

Walk for two to three minutes, hydrating with water.

Isolations (Calisthenics)

Leg Lifts

Music best suited for these is jazz.

Stand beside chair for leg lifts. Hold on to chair with one hand, bending the inside knee slightly. Lift outside leg to front, side, back and inside. Height is not important.

1. Front leg lift, upper thigh: lift leg comfortably to front without bending knee. Do 12 times. Fig. 27.

2. Side leg lift, outer thigh: lift leg comfortably to outside without bending knee or leaning. Do 12 times. Fig. 28.

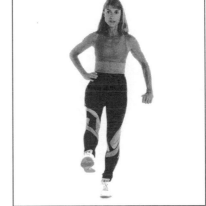

Fig 27

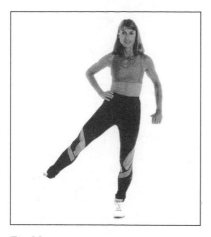

Fig 28

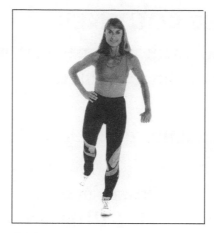

Fig 29

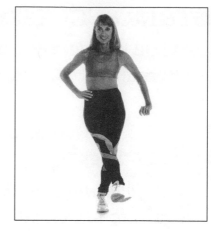

– *Fig 30*

3. Back leg lift, upper back of leg: lean forward slightly, lift leg to back comfortably without bending knee. Do 12 times. Fig. 29.

4. Inner leg lift,inner thigh: sweep leg, crossing inside leg without bending knee. Do 12 times. Change to other side of chair and use opposite leg. Fig. 30.

    Now have a seat, please.

Stretch:

1. Sit tall. Lift right knee to chest. Hold for 12 counts. Lift left knee and hold for 12 counts.

2. Turn to the right, lift left leg to back, hold ankle if it is comfortable. Do not force a stretch. Hold for 12 counts. Turn to left and repeat. Fig. 31.

    Breathe. Take one deep breath, inhaling through nostrils, exhaling through mouth.

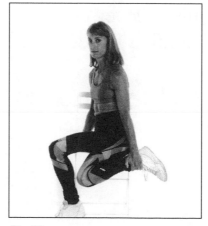

Fig 31

Pelvic Squeezes (Kegels)

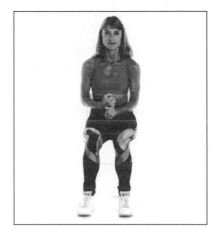

For strengthening urinary tract, stomach and buttock muscles. This may help to prevent incontinence:

1. Sit tall.

2. Squeeze buttocks together tightly and release. Don't be too tense. Imagine trying to hold back a bowel movement by tightening the ring of muscles around the anus. Fig. 32.

Fig 32

3. Repeat this sequence for the length of the music or at your individual discretion.

   Stretch: Sit tall. Lift right knee to chest. Hold for 12 counts. Change legs and repeat.

   Breathe. Take one deep breath, inhaling through nostrils, exhaling through mouth.

Stomach

1. Sit tall.

2. Hold chair with both hands. Lift legs and begin bicycling legs in front. Do this for 12 revolutions. Imagine stomach is against back of chair. Fig. 33.

3. Lift legs, knees bent. Push both legs to front, exhaling through mouth and inhaling through nostrils as legs are pulled into chest. Do 12 times. Fig. 34.

   Stretch. Sit tall. Lift right knee to chest, holding with both hands for the count of 12. Change legs and repeat.

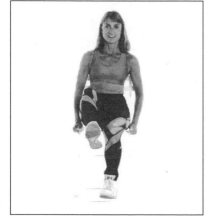

Fig 33

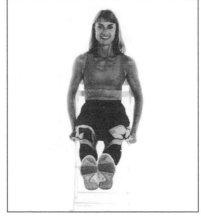

Fig 34

Cool Down Stretches

Limbering, stretching and cooling the muscle is the purpose of the cool down. This routine is essential for a safe, injury-free workout. A slow, gradual, holding set of stretches are being used to bring back the muscles to their pre-exercise position. The music should be slow and easy, lasting five to ten minutes.

Hands

1. Bring each finger to each thumb. Do 6 times. Fig. 35.

2. Bring each finger to the palm. Do 6 times. Fig. 36.

3. Bring thumbs to palms. Do 12 times. Fig. 37.

4. Make a fist, then open fingers and thumbs—wide and straight, in and out. Do 12 times. Fig. 38.

5. Circle hands, 6 to the right and 6 to the left. Fig. 39.

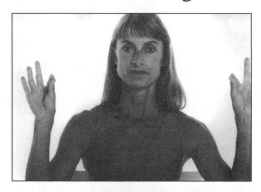

Fig 35

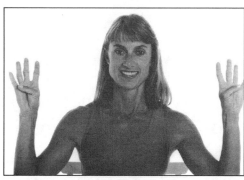

Fig 36

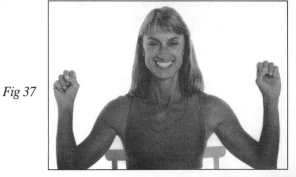

Fig 37

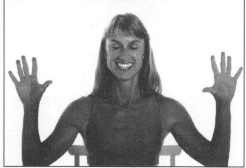

Fig 38

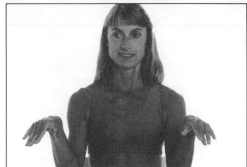

Fig 39

Arms, Shoulders, Upper Back

1. With arms straight out to sides, stretch back and forth from right to left. Do 6 times.

2. Raise both arms in the air; stretch one arm at a time, in a reaching motion. Do 6 times. Lace fingers with palms turned outward. Hold for count of 12. Figs. 40 & 41.

3. Raise both arms to the front, stretching one at a time. Do 6 times. Lace fingers with palms turned outward. Hold for count of 12.

4. Reach one arm down center of back with other arm reaching up until fingers are clasped. Hold for count of 12. Change arm position and repeat. Fig. 42.

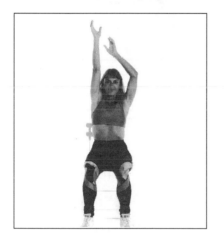

Fig 40

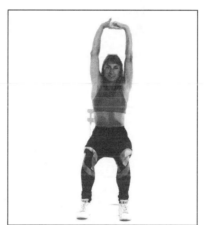

Fig 41

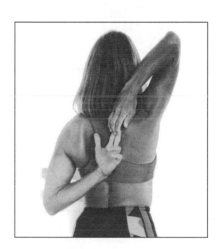

Fig 42

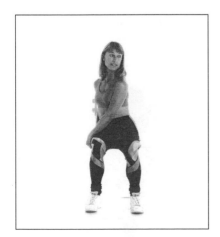

Fig 43

Waist

1. Place right arm down at side. Lean to right and hold front leg of chair, left arm going overhead, for count of 12. Repeat the same on left side.

2. Turn upper torso, from the waist, toward your right. Look over left shoulder, only with your head. Hold for count of 12. Repeat with left turn of upper torso and head turned to right. Fig. 43.

Legs, Stomach

1. Lift the right leg, holding with laced fingers. Point the toe and hold for count of 12. Fig. 44 (No. 1-3).

2. Flex or flatten same foot, and hold for count of 12.

3. Turn the foot to the right, then left, 6 times.

4. Bend knee to chest, hold with hands and circle foot to right 6 times and left 6 times. Place foot on floor and repeat the same with left leg. Fig. 45.

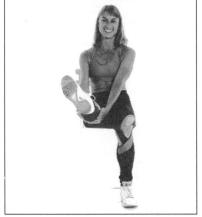

Fig 44

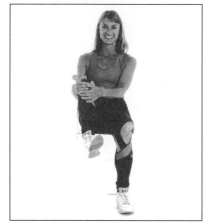

Fig 45

Body Roll

1. Reach out with both arms to front and then as far to floor as possible. Do three rolls and then hold body in limp position toward floor. Close eyes, relax and hold for count of 12. Slowly roll up, keeping head down and eyes closed.

2. Slowly lift both shoulders, 6 times.

3. Slowly roll head to right and left. Keep head forward. Do not roll to back. Roll head back to center and slowly raise head and open eyes. Figs. 46 & 47.

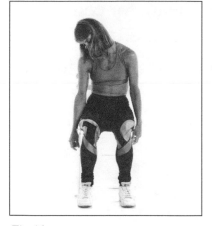

Fig 46

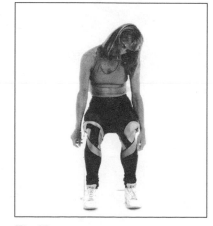

Fig 47

2

WATER (POOL) EXERCISES

WATER (POOL) EXERCISES

THE MUSCLES ARE RELIEVED of normal body pressure in water, and the bones and joints do not have to sustain the weight of the body. Water exercising is especially beneficial for people suffering from arthritis and degenerative diseases. Also, because water is by nature soothing and relaxing, exercising in water is often favored by people who otherwise find exercise unappealing. The body is 10% of its weight in water. The ideal temperature for water when exercising is 84°.

Warm-up: Aquatic Walking

Music for the warm-up should be lively, with an upbeat tempo for walking; three minutes in length.

Remember to keep your body submerged at least up to your waist. Chest deep is best, for at that point the level of difficulty is greatest. Aquatic exercises are effective because of the resistance given by the water. *The purpose of the warm-up is to get muscles lubricated, to stimulate your circulation and prevent stiffness.*

1. Walk forward in water several times back and forth across shallow end. Arms should move the water and steps should be long. Fig. 48.

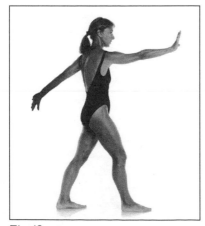
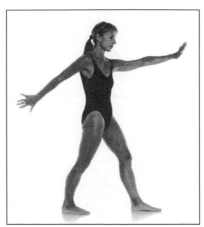
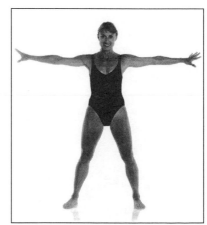

Fig 48   *Fig 49*   *Fig 50*

2. Walk backward in water several times back and forth across shallow end. Move arms back while walking, moving the water. Fig. 49.

3. Walk sideways in water several times back and forth across shallow end. Move arms out to the sides and then together. Fig. 50.

4. Walk to center of pool.

Breathe. Take three deep breaths, inhaling through nose, exhaling through mouth.

Isolations (Calisthenics)

Stretch: Stand in at least waist-deep water unless you are hesitant about being in water. In that case, stand where you are comfortable.

Music should not be as fast as for the walk.

Legs and Feet

Place feet shoulder's-width apart, with pelvis tucked and knees slightly bent. Arms are at sides where it is most comfortable to balance. The area being worked should be submerged in water.

Toe lift for lower front leg:

1. Raise right toes, then return to floor and change to left toes. Do 12 times.

2. Raise both right and left toes together and return to floor. Do 12 times.

Heel lift for lower back leg:

1. From same position as above, raise right heel, return to floor and change to left heel. Do 12 times.

2. Raise both right and left heels together and return to floor. Do 12 times. Fig. 51.

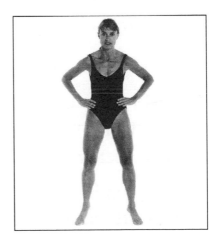

Fig 51

Lunge and lift for lower back of leg and lower front of leg:

1. Place right leg in front of left, a healthy strides distance apart and arms where it is comfortable to balance. Lunge forward slightly with right knee bent, left leg is straight. Both heels are flat. This produces a stretch of the lower back of left leg. Lunge only as far as the stretch is comfortable. Return to upright position. Do 12 times.

2. Next, raise toes from same position and return to floor. Do 12 times. Reverse to left leg. Your upper body should be kept straight while this exercise is performed.

3. Repeat this sequence for the length of the music or at your individual discretion.

   Breathe. Take one deep breath, inhaling through nostrils, exhaling through mouth.

Holding stretches for legs and feet:

1. Put right foot in front of left foot, making sure you can feel the muscle in the lower back of the left leg gently stretch. Lean forward slightly with right knee bent and left leg straight. Keep both heels flat. Hold for 12 counts. See Fig. 70, pg. 34.

2. Next, shift weight backwards, bending left knee and straightening right leg. Hold for 12 counts. Reverse leg positions and repeat.

Squats for upper front of legs:

1. Stand with feet apart, shoulders' width. Turn toes outward with pelvis lifted. Let arms stay comfortably at sides for balance.

2. Keeping buttocks tucked, bend both knees and squat halfway down without leaning forward. Do 12 times. Fig. 52.

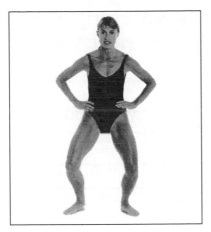

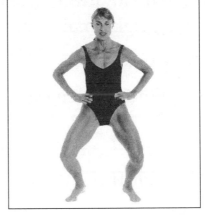

Fig 52   *Fig 53*

3. Lift both heels, keeping them up as you squat halfway down. Continue to keep the buttocks tucked and do not lean forward. Do 12 times. Fig. 53.

4. Repeat sequence for length of music or at your individual discretion.

Holding stretches for upper front of legs:

Raise right arm in air. Bend left knee, lift to rear up to buttocks. Hold, with or without left hand, only if comfortable. Change arm and leg and repeat.

Breathe. Take one deep breath, inhaling through nostrils, exhaling through mouth.

Waist

1. With both arms at sides, shoulders back and feet apart shoulders' width, lean slightly to right, extending arm to right knee while left hand comes up to the waist. Do 12 times. Repeat sequence on left side. See Fig. 72, pg. 35.

2. Hands on shoulders, head facing forward, turn to the right slightly and then to the left, moving water with elbows. Do 12 times. See Fig. 7, pg. 4.

3. Raise both arms in the air, lace fingers. Move arms slightly to the right and then to the left. Do 12 times. See Fig. 73, pg. 35.

4. Stand with left hand behind neck, elbow open, right arm at side. Lean to right with right hand going down to right knee. Do 12 times. Change arms and do 12 times. See Fig. 74, pg. 35.

5. Repeat sequence for length of music or at your individual discretion.

Holding stretch: Lean slightly to right, placing right hand on right knee and left arm over head. Hold for 12 counts. Change sides and repeat.

Breathe. Take one deep breath, inhaling through nostrils and exhaling through mouth.

Arms, Chest, Shoulders, Upper Back

Music is more upbeat for arms than for legs and waist.

Bend down, covering shoulders in water and keeping arms submerged in water. You want to resist the water; always push it away. Get the most benefit from the exercises. For more resistance, strap to your arms a pair of children's water wings or hold jugs filled with water.

1. **Upper front of arms:** Extend arms forward, with hands cupped and wrists tight. Pull right arm to chest, then left arm. Do 12 times. Next, pull both arms together to chest. Do 12 times. See Fig. 11, pg. 6.

2. **Upper back of arms:** With loose fists at chest, extend right arm straight behind, pushing water and lifting arm. Then extend left arm behind. Do 12 times. Remember to keep arms in the water. Next, extend both arms back at the same time. Do 12 times. See Fig. 15, pg. 6.

3. **Chest and shoulders:** Keeping arms submerged in water, bend elbows and cross arms in front. Alternate right over left, then left over right, pushing the water. Do 12 times. Figs. 54 & 55.

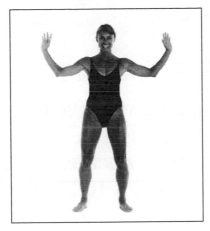

Fig 54

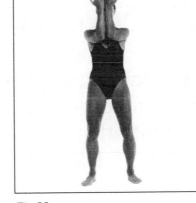

Fig 55

4. **Upper back and shoulders:** Under water, extend arms straight out at sides, keeping fists loose. Bend elbows and push them simultaneously in front of body, then extend them straight out at sides. Do 12 times. See Figs. 16 & 17, pg. 7.

Holding stretches:

1. For shoulders and upper back of arms: Stand up straight and raise both arms above head. Stretch. Next, drop one arm behind head, placing one hand on opposite shoulder, other hand on elbow. Hold for 12. Change arms and repeat sequence.
   See Fig. 18, pg. 8.

2. For upper front of arms: Extend arms out to sides, with palms facing front and slightly toward back. Hold for 12 counts.

3. For upper back: Lace fingers behind back, raise arms and hold for count of 12. See Fig. 19, pg. 8.

4. For chest: Wrap arms around in front, give self a hug and hold for count of 12.

5. Roll shoulders forward 3 times and backward 3 times.

   Breathe. Take three deep breaths, inhaling through nostrils and exhaling slowly through mouth.

Aerobics

Music tempo should be increased so that you can perform the following exercises at a quicker pace.

If you are not comfortable performing any of the following routines, walk back and forth in the shallow end of the pool, increasing to a jog. Remember that aerobic exercise is geared to the cardio-respiratory system. It should be continuous for 10-20 minutes, using the water for resistance. NOTE: The water becomes heavy and you must continually push it, or it may push you into deeper water. You should be submerged in chest deep water. Have a good time. Give 100%!

FIRST ROUTINE

March

1. Lift knees up and down, bringing feet off the floor while alternating legs. Keep floor position of feet close together for count of 12. Repeat with feet further apart for count of 12. Vary the march. Swing arms with hands to opposite shoulders. Vary the arms as you march by orchestrating the arms, as though you are leading a band. Keep arms submerged.

2. March in place, move arms in water, then begin marching forward, backward, right and left.

3. Repeat sequence until the music is finished or at your individual discretion.

SECOND ROUTINE

1. Lift knees while alternating legs. At the same time, raise arms and bring right elbow to left knee. Alternate with left elbow to right knee. Do 12 times. Fig. 56.

2. Kick legs to sides, one at a time, while pushing arms to opposite side of leg kick. Do 12 times. See Fig. 23, pg. 10. Keep arms in water so there is movement. Be sure you lift the legs as you kick to each side.

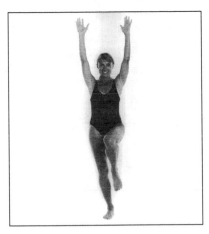
Fig 56

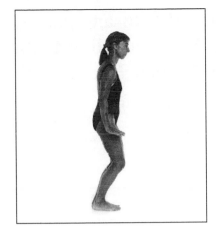
Fig 57

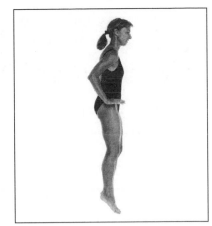
Fig 58

3. Hop forward to wall bending knees together and lifting feet off floor. Push arms down so that the water is being pushed downward. Turn and hop to other wall. Do 3 times. Figs. 57 & 58.

4. Repeat sequence for length of music or at your individual discretion.

THIRD ROUTINE

1. Kick legs forward, one at a time. Simultaneously alternate arms, circling, as in the water crawl. Do 12 times. See Fig. 24, pg. 10.

2. Tap heels while alternating legs. At the same time, push arms forward in water and then back to chest. Do 12 times. See Fig. 25, pg. 10.

3. Kick legs to each side while swinging arms in the same direction in the water. Do 12 times. See Fig. 26, pg. 10.

4. Repeat sequence at your individual discretion.

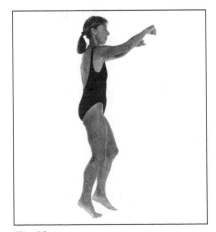
Fig 59

OTHER SUGGESTED ROUTINES

1. Jog forward to the wall and turn. Jogging to the other side, push your arms in the water, alternating with left and right. Do 3 times. Fig. 59.

2. Skip forward to wall and turn and skip to other side. Push arms in water—alternating with left and right. Do 3 times. Fig. 60.

3. Repeat sequence for length of music or at your individual discretion.

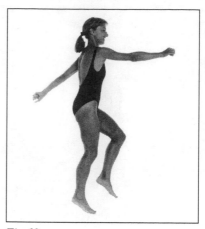

Fig 60

Cool-down Walk

Walk calmly from wall to wall, gently pushing arms for 2 or 3 minutes.

Wall Exercises: Isolations (Calisthenics)

Music should now have a slower tempo.

Breathe. In chest-deep water, walk to wall and take one deep breath, inhaling through nostrils and exhaling through mouth.

Stomach

1. Place back against wall and anchor arms straight out on ledge. Lift knees to chest and keep buttocks against wall. Imagine stomach pushing against wall. (Discomfort may occur through shoulders at first.) Now bicycle legs one at a time. Do 12 times.

2. In same position as above, bring knees to chest. Keeping legs together, push them forward. Do 12 times.

3. In same position, again bring knees to chest. Keeping legs together and buttocks against wall, slowly roll to right, then to left. Do 12 times. This works the sides or waist, as well as the stomach.

4. Repeat sequence for length of music or at your individual discretion.

Stretch: Arms above head. Lift right knee to chest and down. Lift left knee to chest and down. Roll shoulders. Fig. 61.

Breathe. Take one deep breath, inhaling through nostrils, exhaling through mouth.

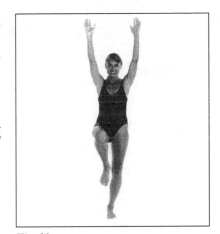

Fig 61

Upper back of legs and buttocks

For buttocks and upper back of legs:

Music should remain at same tempo.

1. Face wall and hold on to it with both hands. Stand up straight with feet together. Lift right leg backward comfortably, without leaning forward and without bending knee. Do not arch back. Do 12 times. Repeat with left leg. Fig. 62.

2. Lift right knee to chest, then extend leg backward, straightening it as the water is being pushed. Do 12 times. Repeat with left leg. Fig. 63.

3. Repeat sequence for length of music or at your individual discretion.

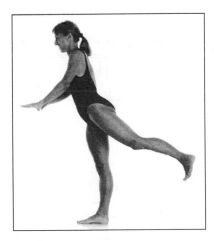

Fig 62

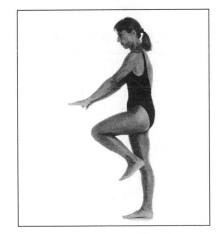

Fig 63

Stretch: Arms above head. Lift right knee to chest, and down, Lift left knee to chest and down.

Breathe. Take one deep breath inhaling through nostrils, exhaling through mouth.

Additional Wall Exercises

Stomach

Face wall and place both hands on wall ledge. Bring both feet up to touch center of wall, bending knees. Keeping legs together, push backward and then bring feet back to wall, as quickly as possible. Do 12 times.

Buttocks, Upper Back of Legs

1. Facing wall, place both hands on wall ledge with elbows pressed to wall—under water. Lift both legs to surface of water. Back should be flat, with no arch. Keeping legs straight, kick them one at a time, under water. Do 12 times. Be careful legs do not lower from the surface of water.

2. From same position, kick legs together, bending knees slightly. Do 12 times.

3. From same position, take legs apart and bring back together, crossing ankles. Do 12 times.

Cool-down Stretches

Limbering, stretching and cooling the muscle is the purpose of the cool down. This routine is essential for a safe, injury-free workout. A slow, gradual, holding set of stretches are being used to bring back the muscles to their pre-exercise condition. Music should be slow and easy.

Legs, Feet, Stomach

1. Face wall, holding on to wall with right hand. Lift left knee to chest and circle ankle 6 times to right, 6 times to left. Fig. 64.

2. Extend same leg to back, stretching gently, and hold for 12 counts. Fig. 65.

3. Extend same leg to front—placing foot on wall at an angle. Straighten leg as best you can; height of leg is not important. Gently stretch. Hold for 12 counts. Fig. 66.

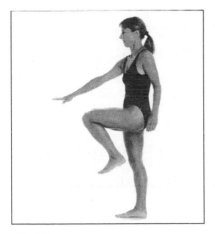
Fig 64

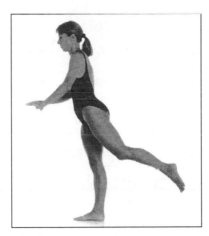
Fig 65

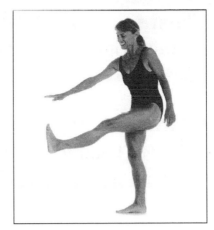
Fig 66

4. Placc foot on floor, and hold wall with left hand. Lift right knee to chest and repeat sequence as above (Nos. 1-3). (Circles lubricate joints; leg extensions gently lengthen muscles.

Hands

1. Drop hands from wall. Walk backward 3 steps. Keep hands in water. Bring each finger to thumb 6 times and each finger to palm 6 times. Figs. 35-37, pg. 14.

2. Make a fist, then extend fingers and thumbs—wide and straight, in and out. Do 12 times. Fig. 38, pg. 14.

3. Circle hands 6 times right and 6 left. Fig. 39, pg. 14.

Arms, Shoulders, Chest, Upper Back

1. Face front. Turn to right from the waist up, looking over left shoulder. Hold for 12 counts. Turn to left in same manner.

2. Raise arms above head—stretching arms one at a time, 6 times. Lace fingers and hold for 12 counts. Lean slightly to right and to left. Do 6 times. Figs. 40 & 41, pg. 15.

3. Stretch arms one at a time right to left, 6 times. Hold arms straight out from sides for 12 count.

4. With arms down at sides, lift shoulders up and down slowly. Do 6 times.

Waist

Raise right arm in air — lean to left and hold for 12 count. Change sides and repeat.

Head rolls

Lower head forward. Do not roll to back. Close your eyes and slowly roll head to right and slowly to left. Now back to center and raise.

GOOD JOB!

3

INDOOR STANDING

AND

FLOOR EXERCISES

INDOOR STANDING AND FLOOR EXERCISES

THESE EXERCISES ARE CONDUCTED while in a standing position for the first thirty minutes. The next twenty minutes are from the floor. A mirrored wall, although unnecessary, would be advantageous, enabling you to watch your form. Using a towel or mat would allow you to be more comfortable while on the floor. The ideal temperature for exercising indoors in 74°.

Warm-up

Warm-up exercises serve to increase the heart rate and blood circulation slowly. When muscles are warm and joints lubricated, the body can respond to movement with greater flexibility. Warming up is also an essential step in preventing injury.

Breathe. Take three deep breaths, inhaling through the nostrils and exhaling slowly through the mouth.

Warm-up Exercises:

Music should have an upbeat tempo, but not too fast, lasting approximately 3 minutes.

Begin your warm-up by standing in a relaxed position with pelvis lifted, knees bent slightly.

1. Point the right toe, raise both arms in the air on right side; bring right foot back and point the left toe, lowering arms to waist. Do 12 times. Fig. 67.

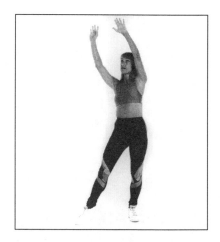

Fig 67

2. Tap right heel, then left, alternating as both arms are pushing forward. Do 12 times. See Fig. 2, pg. 3.

3. Lift right knee, then left, alternating knee lifts and taking both arms to right and then left according to the knee being lifted. You can always vary this by moving arms to the opposite side of the knee lift. Do 12 times. See Fig. 3, pg. 3.

4. Do this sequence for the length of the music chosen or at your individual discretion.

It should be noted that if an exercise does not feel comfortable, either it should be eliminated from the workout or repetitions should be decreased. Also, if a physically limited person is unable to exercise an arm or a leg, adapt the exercises to the capabilities.

Breathe. Take one deep breath, inhaling through nostrils and exhaling slowly through mouth.

Isolations (Calisthenics)

Maintenance of strength is of great importance to living better and more independently. This segment begins with isolations of specific muscles, to build strength. For all of the following, it is important always to stand with pelvis lifted, stomach and buttocks tucked in, shoulders back and head held up. In some of these exercises you may feel more secure holding on to a window ledge or chair.

Music should have a beat somewhat slower than for warm-up. Listening to favorite songs makes the program more fun and enjoyable.

Legs and Feet

1. Toe lift for lower front of legs: Stand with feet apart at shoulders' width. Place hands on hips or down at sides. Raise the right toes and return to floor. Raise the left toes and return to floor. Do 12 times. Next, raise right and left toes together and return to floor. Do 12 times. Fig. 68.

2. Heel lift for lower back of legs: Stand with feet apart at shoulders' width. Raise right heel and return to floor. Repeat with left heel. Do 12 times. Fig. 69.

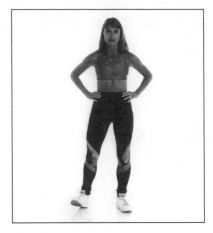

Fig 68

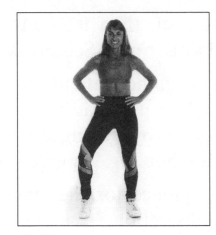

Fig 69

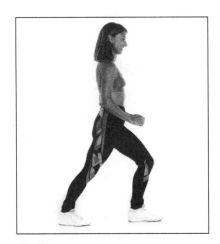

Fig 70

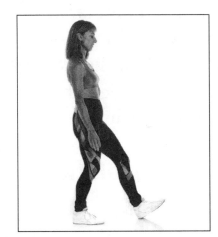

Fig 71

3. Lunge and lift for lower back and lower front of legs: With arms held out from sides, place right foot a stride's length in front of left. Lunge forward slightly, with right knee bent, left leg straight, both heels flat. Lunge only as far as the stretch is comfortable. Return to upright position. Do 12 times. Fig. 70.

4. Retain position. Raise right toes, then return to floor. Do 12 times. Reverse exercise, lunging with left leg. Upper body should be straight while this exercise is performed. Fig. 71.

5. Repeat this sequence for the length of music or at your individual discretion.

6. Holding (static stretches): Place right foot a stride's length in front of left, with feet aligned. With right leg bent, lean forward slightly, with hands resting on right knee. Hold for 12 counts. Now bring right

leg back and put left leg forward, bending left knee and straightening right leg. With hands resting on left knee, hold for 12 counts.

Breathe. Take one deep breath inhaling through nostrils and exhaling through mouth.

Waist

For the following exercises, stand with feet apart, at shoulders' width, with pelvis lifted, stomach and buttocks tucked in. Keep hips stationary and forward.

1. With both arms at sides, shoulders back and feet flat on floor, lean slightly to right, extending arm halfway down leg of chair while left hand comes up to the waist. Do 12 times. Repeat sequence on left side. Fig. 72.

2. Hands on shoulders, head facing forward, turn to the right slightly and then to the left. Do 12 times. See Fig. 7, pg. 4.

3. Raise both arms in the air, lace fingers. Move arms slightly to the right and left. Do 12 times. Fig. 73.

4. Repeat for length of music or at your discretion.

5. Static stretch: Lean to right, resting right hand on right knee and left arm over head. Hold for 12 counts. Change to left side. Hold for 12 counts. Fig. 74.

Breathe. Take one deep breath, inhaling through nostrils and exhaling through mouth.

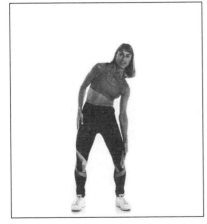
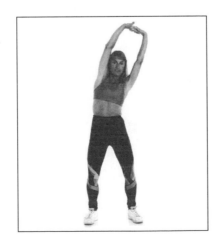
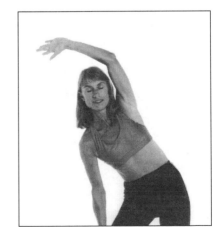

Fig 72 *Fig 73* *Fig 74*

Arms, Chest, Shoulders, Upper Back

For the following exercises, one- or two-pound hand weights (or soup cans) may be used to increase resistance. The weights may be used for sequences 1-7. Assume this posture: Stand with feet apart, at shoulders' width, pelvis lifted, stomach and buttocks tucked in. Lean upper torso forward slightly, with hips stationary and forward.

Upper front of arms:

1. Rest elbows on waist and bring forearms against chest, cupping hands and pressing against the air. Pressing back against chair, lower arms, then raise them back to chest. Do 12 times. See Fig. 10, pg. 5.

2. Extend arms to the front with your forearms facing up and hands cupped. Bring cupped hands to shoulders pressing against the air. Do 12 times. See Fig. 11, pg. 6.

Upper back of arms:

1. With arms extended straight up, lace fingers and squeeze elbows to head. Take both arms behind head, as far down as possible, bending the elbows but keeping them close to the head, then raising arms in the air above head. Avoid over-extension into face area. Do 12 times. See Figs. 12 & 13, pg. 6.

2. Place hands on each side of chest, make loose fists, bend elbows. Extend arms behind and then return to sides of chest. Do 12 times. See Figs. 14 & 15, pg. 6.

Chest and shoulders:

Bend both elbows with forearms extended in air on each side of chest. Bring both arms together, elbow to elbow, then back to the sides. Do 12 times. See Figs. 54 & 55, pg. 23.

Upper back and shoulders:

1. Extend arms straight out from sides, with loose fists. Bend elbows, bringing arms in front of chest, fists coming together. Do 12 times. See Figs. 16 & 17, pg. 7.

2. Repeat sequence until music is finished or at your individual discretion.

Static or holding stretches:

The following stretches can be done from a standing position or in a chair.

1. For upper back of arms and shoulders: Raise arms above head, dropping one arm behind head, placing one hand on opposite shoulder, other hand on elbow. Hold for a count of 12. Change arms and do the same for holding count of 12. See Fig. 18, pg. 8.

2. For upper front of arms: Extend arms to sides with palms facing front and slightly toward back. Hold for a count of 12.

3. For upper back: Lace fingers behind back, raise arms and hold for a count of 12. See Fig. 19, pg. 8.

4. For chest: Wrap arms around in front, give self a hug and hold for a count of 12.

5. Raise arms in air, bend knees and keep them bent as you roll as close to the floor as you can. Roll up slowly.

6. Roll shoulders forward three times and backward three times. Shake out arms, legs, and body.

Breathe. Take three deep breaths, inhaling through nostrils and exhaling through mouth.

Low Impact Aerobics

These exercises, which are geared to the cardio-respiratory system, strengthen the heart and lungs. Because the heart is a muscle, it requires exercise to keep it toned and healthy. And the healthier the heart, the more efficiently the blood is pumped throughout the body. As the health of the lungs improves, the circulation of oxygen expands, and cells, tissues and muscles are better nourished. This builds endurance. *Low impact* refers to one foot always on the floor. It should be noted that if any exercise does not feel comfortable it should be eliminated from the workout. Give 100%!

Music for these routines should be increased in tempo so that exercises will be performed at a quicker pace. Use three different songs lasting ten to twenty minutes in total. Have fun!

FIRST ROUTINE

1. March: Lift knees up and down, bringing feet off the floor while alternating legs. Keep floor position of feet close together for count of 12. Repeat with feet further apart for count of 12. Vary the march. Swing arms with hands to opposite shoulders. Vary the arms as you march by orchestrating the arms, as though you are leading a band. Then raise arms in the air and wave. This can be performed in a standing position. While marching, vary the march by moving forward, backwardd, right and left. Be sure knees are lifted high and arms are moving.

2. Repeat sequence until the music is finished or at your individual discretion.

SECOND ROUTINE

1. Lift knees while alternating legs. At the same time, raise arms and bring right elbow to left knee. Alternate with left elbow to right knee. Do 12 times. See Fig. 22, pg. 10.

2. Kick legs to sides, one at a time, while pushing arms to opposite side of leg kick. Do 12 times. While doing the routine, remember you can add a hop for impact and you can always go forward, backward, right and left to keep it fun and interesting. See Fig. 23, pg. 10.

3. Hop forward 3 times, bending knees together and lifting feet off floor. Push arms forward. Hop backward 3 times using same positioning. Repeat sequence 3 times. See Figs. 57 & 58, pg. 25.

4. Repeat sequence until music is finished or at your individual discretion.

THIRD ROUTINE

1. Kick legs forward, one at a time. Simultaneously alternate arms, circling, as in the water crawl. Do 12 times. See Fig. 24, pg. 10.

2. Tap heels while alternating legs. At the same time, push arms forward and then back to chest. Do 12 times. See Fig. 25, pg. 10.

3. Kick legs to each side while swinging arms in the same direction. Do 12 times. While doing the routine, remember you can add a hop for impact and you can always go forward, backward, right and left to keep it fun and interesting. See Fig. 26, pg. 10.

4. Repeat sequence until music is finished or at your individual discretion.

Cool Down Walk

Walk for 2-3 minutes, hydrating with water. When you feel cooled down, get your mat or towel and lie on the floor and relax. Stretch out long and be sure you have enough room to move about comfortably.

Floor Exercises: Isolations (Calisthenics)

Music for the beginning floor stretch and stomach tightening should have a good tempo—not too fast, not too slow. Jazz is good!

Remember with the following exercises your form is *very* important. You can always increase repetitions when your work-out becomes more familiar and consistent. The muscles should fatigue or slightly tire. Enjoy toning your many muscles!

Stretch

Extend your arms behind your head, with your legs extended long and flat—point toes, flatten or flex feet. Do 12 times. Fig. 75.

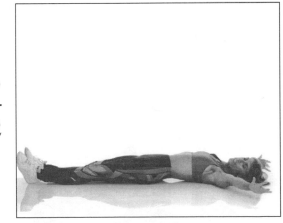

Fig 75

Facial Exercises

Lie with arms at sides, legs flat.

1. Move mouth from right to left with head resting on floor. Do 12 times. Fig. 76.

2. Move jaw forward and back. Do 12 times. Fig. 77.

3. Stick tongue in and out of mouth. Do 12 times. Fig. 78.

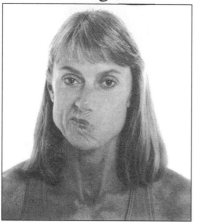
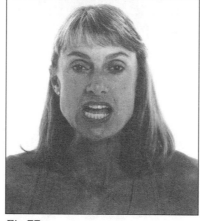
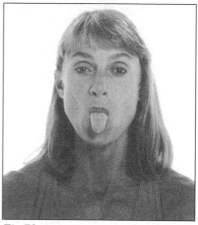

Fig 76   *Fig 77*   — *Fig 78*

Pushups

1. Roll to one side. Lift up on one elbow and then on hands. Stack hips and curl up legs away from arms. Push chest to floor keeping chin in line with chest. Keep elbow off floor and now lift up. Do 12 times. Figs. 79 & 80.

2. Change sides, placing hands close together to do push-up. Do 12 times.

The closer the hands are together, the more the upper back of arm is worked; the farther apart the hands, the more the chest is worked. This is a very good upper body strengthener.

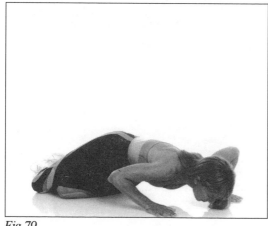
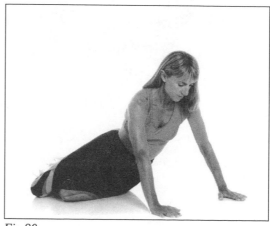

Fig 79   *Fig 80*

Stretch:

1. Sit tall and stretch arms above head. Hold for 12 counts.
2. Place both arms down center of back, bending elbows and keeping them opened. Hold for 12 counts.
3. Wrap arms around self and give hug. Hold for 12 counts.
4. Roll shoulders forward 3 times and backward 3 times.

   Breathe. Take one deep breath, inhaling through nostrils, exhaling through mouth.

   Now lie down.

Stomach

1. Bend both knees, with feet and back flat on floor and finger tips on head. *Elbows can be opened or closed. Opened elbow is flat, closed is to head. Opened elbow is more difficult than a closed elbow.* Lift chest and shoulders off floor to point of a contraction; return chest and shoulders to floor. Do 12 times. *This works upper part of stomach.* Avoid unnecessary head motion; exhale through mouth as you lift and inhale through nostrils as you lower. Fig. 81.

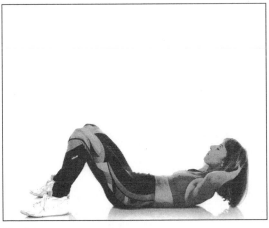

Fig 81

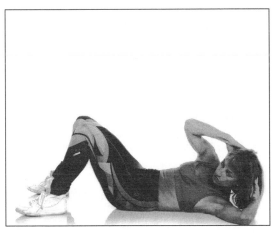

Fig 82

2. Bend both knees, with feet and back flat on floor and finger tips on head. Lift right shoulder as the right elbow reaches toward left knee. Keep left shoulder flat on floor. Do 12 times. Change to left shoulder and elbow to right knee. Do 12 times. *This works the inner part of*

stomach and sides. Inhale through nostrils as you lift and exhale through mouth as you lower. Fig. 82.

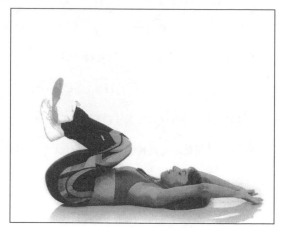

3. Bend knees and lift feet off floor. Extend arms behind head. Keeping lower back flat, lift buttocks off floor, pressing stomach down as buttocks are lifted. Return buttocks to floor. Do 12 times. *This works the lower part of stomach.* Fig. 83.

Fig 83

4. Repeat sequence until music is finished or at your individual discretion.

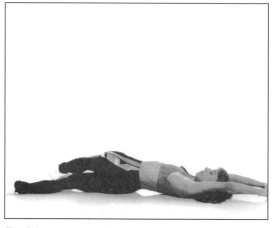

Fig 84

Stretch: Legs out flat, with arms extended behind head. Stretch long. Roll slightly to right and stretch, then roll slightly to left and stretch. Roll to center. Fig. 84.

Breathe. Take one deep breath, inhaling through nostrils, exhaling through mouth.

Outer Thighs

Music for this should have a little faster tempo than that for the stomach tightener.

1. Lie on left side. Left arm can either be extended on floor with head resting on it, or elbow can bend and you can rest weight on forearm, with head up. In this case, both hands will be on floor in front of body. Stack hips and curl up left leg for balance.

2. Bend right knee, then lift right leg half way. Do 12 times. Fig. 85.

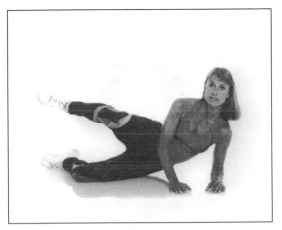

Fig 85

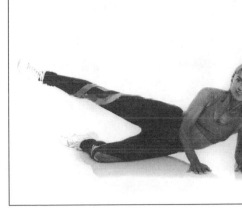

Fig 86

3. Extend right leg out. Avoid locking the knee tight. Lift leg half way up, parallel to lower leg. Do 12 times. Fig. 86.

4. Lift extended leg half way up and bring knee to chest and extend leg 12 times.

5. Repeat sequence at individual discretion. Repeat all of above on opposite side.

Stretch: Lying on back, bend both knees and lift to chest. Place right foot on left knee and gently stretch. Count to 12. Change legs and stretch. Count to 12.

NOTE: The leg extended or parallel is always a little more difficult to lift than a bent knee.

Inner Thighs

Music for this is about the same tempo as for the outer thigh.

1. Lying on back, bring both knees to chest. Place hands under hips to help keep legs up. Fig. 87.

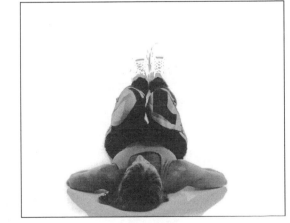

Fig 87

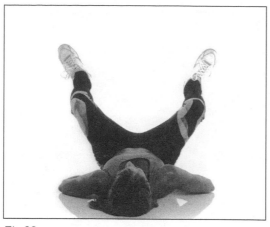

Fig 88

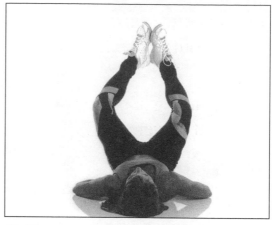

Fig 89

2. Take legs apart and bring back together, with knees and ankles going apart and together at same time. Do 12 times. Fig. 88.

3. With knees bent and at chest, take knees and ankles apart for a double count. Do 12 times. Fig. 88.

4. With knees bent and at chest, keep feet together and take knees apart. Do 12 times. Fig. 89.

5. Repeat sequence for length of music or at your individual discretion.

   Stretch: With knees bent, place bottoms of feet together. Hold ankles and gently stretch for 12 counts.

   NOTE: While doing the exercises 1-5 above, legs can be extended straight up in the air. This makes them more difficult.

Upper Front of Legs

Music should be at about the same tempo as for the outer and inner thigh.

1. Sit up, then rest weight on elbows. Bend left knee. Lift right leg half way up, then down. Repeat 12 times. Fig. 90.

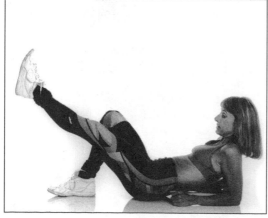

Fig 90

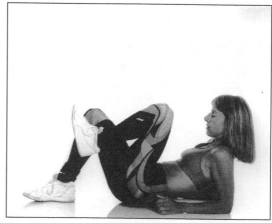

Fig 91

2. Bend right knee and bring to chest, then extend leg out to front. Do 12 times. Fig. 91.

3. Extend right leg and lift half way up and pulse (slight movement without dropping leg) to count of 12. Fig. 92.

4. With opposite legs, repeat sequence.

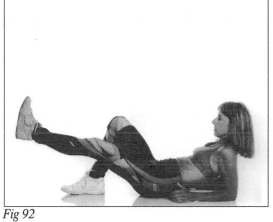
Fig 92

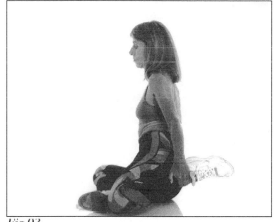
Fig 93

Stretch: Sit up and bend right knee, holding ankle if possible. *However, do not force stretch.* Lean slightly to left and gently stretch. Hold for 12 counts. Reverse and repeat sequence. Fig. 93.

NOTE: if it is too tiring or uncomfortable to be on elbows, sit upright. *Do not lie flat.*

Buttocks, Upper Back of Legs

Music tempo should now increase a little.

1. Lie on back. With arms down at sides, bend knees and keep feet, lower back and head flat on floor. Slowly lift pelvis up two inches off floor and squeeze buttocks together tightly. Lift up and down 12 times, squeezing tightly as buttocks are lifted. Be sure to keep lower back on floor. Fig. 94.

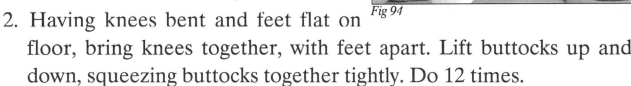
Fig 94

2. Having knees bent and feet flat on floor, bring knees together, with feet apart. Lift buttocks up and down, squeezing buttocks together tightly. Do 12 times.

3. With feet flat on floor, bent knees can be either together or apart. Lift buttocks; pulse (slight movement without dropping buttocks to floor) to count of 12.

Stretch: Bring knees to chest, with arms underneath legs and fingers laced. Gently stretch and hold for count of 12.

NOTE: This works three sets of muscles: 1) buttocks, 2) upper back of legs, 3) urinary tract.

Breathe. Take one deep breath, inhaling through nostrils, exhaling through mouth.

Cool Down Stretches

Limbering, stretching and cooling the muscles is the purpose of the cool down. This routine is essential for a safe, injury-free workout. A slow, gradual, holding set of stretches are being used to bring back the muscles to their pre-exercise condition.

Music should be a slow and easy tempo.

Hands (Figs. 35 - 39, pg. 14.)

1. Lie back, extending legs out flat. Raise forearms, keeping elbows on floor. Bring each finger to thumb, one at a time. Do 6 times.

2. Bring each finger to palm, one at a time. Do 6 times.

3. Bring thumbs to palm. Do 6 times.

4. Make a fist and extend fingers and thumbs wide and straight—in and out. Do 12 times.

5. Circle hands or wrists—6 times to right and 6 times to left. *Circling lubricates joints.*

6. Rest arms at sides.

Upper Back of Legs

1. Lying flat on floor with arms at sides, bend both knees. Bring right knee to chest and wrap arms around knee. Circle ankle to right 6 times and to left 6 times. Fig. 95.

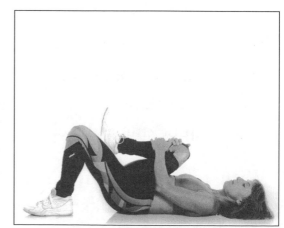

Fig 95

2. Extend leg in air, supporting it with both hands by holding it above back of knee. Gently stretch. Hold for 12 counts. Fig. 96.

3. Repeat with opposite leg.

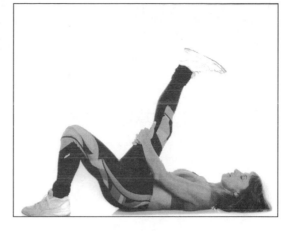

Fig 96

Lower Back

1. Extend legs out flat, with arms out at sides. Cross right leg over left and slowly roll until chest is half way on floor. Hold for 12 counts. Slowly roll to center. Reverse to left leg over right and repeat rolling sequence. Hold for 12 counts. Fig. 97.

2. Lift both knees to chest with legs together. Extend arms out at sides. Slowly roll to the right, head to the left, keeping shoulders flat. Hold for 12 counts. Reverse sequence, slowly rolling to the left, head to the right. Hold for 12 counts. Fig. 98.

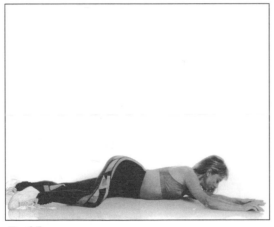

Fig 97

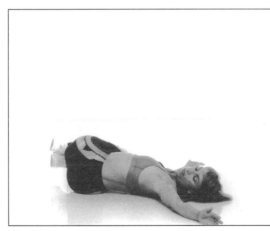

Fig 98

Shoulders

Sit up tall, close eyes and lift shoulders up and down. Do 6 times.

Head Rolls

Sit up tall, close eyes and slowly turn head to right and slowly to left. Do not roll to back. Turn slowly back to center. Figs. 46 & 47, pg. 16.

GOOD JOB!

BIBLIOGRAPHY

Aerobic Theory and Practice. Sherman Oaks, California: AEROBICS AND FITNESS ASSOCIATION OF AMERICA, 1990.

Aerobic-Dance-Exercise Instructor Manual. San Diego, California: INTERNATIONAL DANCE-EXERCISE ASSOCIATION, 1987.

Anderson, Bob. *Stretching*. Bolinas, California: SHELTER PUBLICATIONS, INC., 1980.

Brown, Dawn. "Aqua-Size I Video." Newark, New Jersey: HALLOWELL AND COMPANY, PPI, 1987.

Casey, Maura. "Wheelercize Video." South Bound Brook, New Jersey: SCOTT AND KC ENTERPRISES, 1986.

Katz, Jane. *The W. E. T. Workout*. New York, New York: FACTS ON FILE PUBLICATIONS, 1985.

McKenzie, Robin. *Treat Your Own Back*. New Zealand: SPINAL PUBLICATIONS LTD., 1987.

Switkes, Betty. *Senior-Cize*. Washington, D.C., 1982.

Additional copies of
THE FIFTY MINUTE WORKOUT
FOR PEOPLE OVER FIFTY
by Gaily Warren,
may be ordered by
sending $12.95 postpaid
for each copy to:

DISTINCTIVE PUBLISHING CORP.
P.O. Box 17868
Plantation, FL 33318-7868
305-975-2413

Quantity discounts
are also available
from the publisher